50 Bad Breath Meal Solutions:

Get Rid of Your Bad Breath Problem in Just a Few Days

By

Joe Correa CSN

COPYRIGHT

ACKNOWLEDGEMENTS

This book is dedicated to my friends and family that have had mild or serious illnesses so that you may find a solution and make the necessary changes in your life.

50 Bad Breath Meal Solutions:

Get Rid of Your Bad Breath Problem in Just a Few Days

By

Joe Correa CSN

CONTENTS

ABOUT THE AUTHOR

After years of Research, I honestly believe in the positive effects that proper nutrition can have over the body and mind. My knowledge and experience has helped me live healthier throughout the years and which I have shared with family and friends. The more you know about eating and drinking healthier, the sooner you will want to change your life and eating habits.

Nutrition is a key part in the process of being healthy and living longer so get started today. The first step is the most important and the most significant.

INTRODUCTION

50 Bad Breath Meal Solutions: Get Rid of Your Bad Breath Problem in Just a Few Days

By Joe Correa CSN

We all know that awkward moment when we just can't resist that garlic pasta or a nice bowl of spring salad with onions and people walk away, avoiding contact or even offer us some chewing gum. That is perfectly normal and everyone has experienced that at least once in their lifetime.

However, when these situations become common, then even a simple "face to face" conversation becomes a problem. You're not alone in this. About 3 billion people in the world have what doctors call "halitosis", or a bad breath problem, and it's not some modern disease. People have been dealing with this problem for generations, trying to find a solution because bad breath can affect us in so many ways: our social life, our self confidence when interacting with other people, and everything else that goes with it.

Besides oral hygiene, there are many factors that stimulate bad breath like digestive tract issues, diabetes, respiratory and kidney problems, an unhealthy diet, etc.

Smoking, drinking coffee, stress, specific foods, alcohol, and certain spices, are the main culprits for bad breath. There is really no need for drastic changes to fix this problem, just some simple dietary changes are more than enough to make significant changes in your social life.

Having this in mind, I have created these delicious and healthy recipes with carefully chosen ingredients to help you fight bad breath problems. To enjoy these recipes, you will need plenty of "bad breath super foods" like avocado, apple, citrus fruits, berries, ginger, cumin, etc. These ingredients are proven to help you solve this rather unpleasant feeling. Never again will you have to worry about that business meeting or a date!

I want these recipes to be a guideline to a healthier life for you and your family. That is exactly why I know you will enjoy these recipes! They are tasty, healthy, and contain some powerful ingredients that WILL solve the problem.

With proper oral hygiene and this book, the results are inevitable. Enjoy my special "Ginger Cookies" over a cup of mint tea in the afternoon family gathering. You will notice a huge difference. And if you're a huge garlic fan, you will learn that there is no need to completely avoid it.

You just have to prepare it properly and that specific "garlic breath" will be history.

Meet new people and make friends. Don't let your bad breath stop you starting a new conversation!

50 BAD BREATH MEAL SOLUTIONS: GET RID OF YOUR BAD BREATH PROBLEM IN JUST A FEW DAYS

1. Ginger Cookies

Ingredients:

9 oz of all-purpose flour

2 tsp of ginger, ground

½ tsp of salt

¼ tsp of cinammon

5 oz of butter

1 cup of honey

1 large egg

3 tbsp of honey

Preparation:

Preheat the oven to 350°F.

Combine flour, ginger, salt, and cinammon in a large mixing bowl. Stir well to combine. Set aside

Whisk the egg, butter, and honey. Now, combine both mixtures together and stir all well.

Meanwhile, line some baking paper in a large baking sheet.

Using your hands, form cookie shapes and place into a baking sheet. Bake for 10 minutes and remove from the oven to cool.

You can serve your cookies with some homemade fruit jam, or simply with a glass of milk.

Enjoy!

Nutritional information per serving: Kcal: 123, Protein: 0.9g, Carbs: 19.7g, Fats: 4.2g

2. Cinammon Muffins

Ingredients:

1 cup of all-purpose flour

¼ cup of honey

1 tsp of yeast

1 tbsp of butter, melted

2 cups of skim milk

1 tsp od salt

1 tsp of cinammon, ground

For topping:

2 tbsp of almond, roughly chopped

1 tbsp of butter

1 tbsp of honey

1 tsp of cinammon

Preparation:

Combine dry ingredients in a large bowl and mix well. Now gently stir in 1 tablespoon of melted butter and milk, until the dough forms a ball. You can add some more milk to get the right consistency. Mix well for a few minutes, using your hands or an electric mixer. The dough will become very sticky.

Now add some more flour (2 tablespoons should be enough) to get a nice and smooth mixture. Cover and let it rise for about 15 minutes.

Meanwhile, preheat the oven to 350°F. Use a muffin molds to shape your muffins. Bake for about 20 minutes, until nice gold brown color. Remove from the oven to cool.

Now, combine all topping ingredients in a large skillet over a medium-high temperature. Stir and cook until it all combines, or butter melts. Pour over the topping over muffins and refrigerate for 10 minutes.

Serve!

Nutritional information per serving: Kcal: 145, Protein: 5.2g, Carbs: 28.4g, Fats: 10.2g

3. Avocado Ziti Pesto

Ingredients:

10 oz of ziti pasta,

2 medium-sized avocado, peeled, pit removed, and chopped

1 tsp of fresh basil, finely chopped

1 tsp of pine nuts, chopped (or any other that you have on hand)

½ cup of olive oil

1 tsp of salt

1 tsp of black pepper, ground

1 tbsp of lemon juice

1 tsp of lemon zest

Preparation:

Follow the instructions on the package to cook ziti. Remove after cooking and transfer to serving plate.

Meanwhile, combine basil, pine nuts, avocados, lemon juice, and olive oil in large mixing bowl. Sprinkle with some salt and pepper and stir well to combine. Set the pesto aside.

Pour pesto over the ziti and season with lemon zest on top.

Enjoy!

Nutritional information per serving: Kcal: 447, Protein: 9.8g, Carbs: 48.2g, Fats: 23.1g

4. Beets with Mint Sauce

Ingredients:

2 lb of beets, trimmed and sliced

1 tbsp of olive oil

For dressing:

¼ cup of mint leaves, finely chopped

1 tbsp of lemon juice

1 tsp of honey

½ tsp of salt

Preparation:

Preheat the oven to 400°F.

Wrap beet slices in a greased aluminum foil and place the into the oven. Bake beets for 1 hour, or until soften. Remove from the heat and leave it while to cool.

Meanwhile, combine the dressing ingredients in a mixing bowl and whisk well the mixture.

Transfer beets to the serving plate and drizzle with dressing. Sprinkle with some extra pinch of salt and garnish with some fresh mint leaves.

Nutritional information per serving: Kcal: 82, Protein: 0.2g, Carbs: 2.6g, Fats: 5.1g

5. Warm Chicken Bowl

Ingredients:

1 ½ lb of fire roasted tomatoes, diced

12 chicken thighs, boneless and skinless

1 tbsp of dried basil, ground

8 oz of milk, ful fat

½ tsp of salt

½ tsp of black pepper, ground

7 oz of tomato paste

3 celery stalks, chopped

3 medium-sized carrots, chopped

2 tbsp of olive oil

1 finely chopped onion

4 garlic cloves, minced

½ container of mushrooms

Preparation:

Preheat olive oil in a frying pan over medium-high temperature. Add the celery, onions and carrots and fry for 5 to 10 minutes.

Transfer to the skillet and add tomato paste, basil, garlic, mushrooms and seasoning. Keep stirring the vegetables till they are completely covered by tomato sauce. At the same time, cut the chicken into small cubes to make it easier to eat.

Put the chicken in the skillet, pour the olive oil over it and throw in the tomatoes. Stir the chicken in to ensure the ingredients and vegetables are properly mixed with it. Turn the heat to low and cook for about 30 minutes.

The vegetables and chicken should be cooked completely before you turn the heat off.

Serve

Nutritional information per serving: Kcal: 504, Protein: 36.3g, Carbs: 72.4g, Fats: 6.8g

6. Autumn Soup

Ingredients:

3 medium-sized sweet potatoes, chopped

1 tsp of salt

2 sliced fennel bulbs

15 oz of pureed pumpkin

1 large onion sliced

1 tbsp of olive oil

½ tsp of pumpkin pie spice

50 oz boiling water

Preparation:

Heat up 1 tablespoon of oil ina crock pot over a medium-high temperature.

Now, turn the heat to low and add onion and fennel bulbs. Cover with a lid and continue to cook until caramelized.

Add the rest of the ingredients to the pot and continue cooking till the sweet potatoes are sour. Cook on low heat to get the best possible result. After the process is completed, blend the soup until it is smooth and then add salt to taste.

Enjoy!

Nutritional information per serving: Kcal: 230, Protein: 1.3g, Carbs: 32.6g, Fats: 12.3g

7. Spanish Chicken

Ingredients:

6 chicken thighs, skinless

½ cauliflower head, chopped

1 tsp of salt

1 can of tomatoes, chopped

½ lb of Brussels sprouts

1 medium-sized chorizo sausage

3 medium-sized zucchini, peeled and sliced

2 tbsp of vegetable oil

Preparation:

Take a frying pan and add some oil. Fry the chicken thighs, removing the skin if you want, until they turn golden brown. Remove the thighs from the frying pan and move to a large pot. Next, chop the sausage and fry for around 3 minutes. After frying, put it in the pot as well.

Slice the zucchinis and break the cauliflower into small florets and put them in the pot as well. Also add the Brussels sprouts to the pot. Add salt and then pour the chopped tomatoes over the ingredients. Set the heat to low and cook for about an hour. Serve with a side of baby corn.

Nutritional information per serving: Kcal: 431, Protein: 27.7g, Carbs: 38.4g, Fats: 13.2g

8. White Mushrooms Beef Tips

Ingredients:

2 pounds of grass-fed beef stew meat, cubed

Salt and ground pepper, to taste

2 tablespoons of olive oil

2 cups of fresh white mushrooms

2 cups of beef stock

½ white onion, chopped

1 tablespoon minced garlic

Preparation:

Season the beef with salt and pepper and toss to coat it evenly with spices.

In a stew pot over medium-high heat, add the oil and brown the beef evenly on all sides. Stir in the garlic and onions, sauté for 2 minutes and add the mushrooms

Add the oil in the inner pot, press the sauté button and adjust to brown mode. Season beef with salt and pepper and brown evenly on all sides in the inner pot. Stir in the onions and garlic and sauté for about 1 minute and then add the mushrooms and the stock. Cover with lid, bring it to a boil and reduce to low heat. Simmer for about 30 minutes or until the meat is tender and cooked through.

Adjust the seasoning and transfer into a serving bowl. Serve immediately.

Nutritional information per serving: Kcal: 235, Protein: 28.8g, Carbs: 18.4g, Fats: 7.2g

9. Turkey in Orange Sauce

Ingredients:

2 tbsp of clarified butter

1 lb of turkey breast slices

1 tsp of salt

1 tsp of black pepper, ground

1 cup of chicken stock

2 tablespoons of butter

1 tsp of honey

2 tsp of orange zest

2 tbsp of fresh orange, juiced

1 tsp of Cayenne pepper, ground

Preparation:

Season the slices of turkey evenly with salt and pepper on both sides.

Add the butter into the pan and apply medium-high heat. When the butter melts, brown the turkey meat on both sides and transfer into a plate. Set aside.

Add more butter, orange zest, orange juice, cayenne and the stock in the same pan and cook until it reaches to a simmer. Return the turkey meat in the pan and baste with sauce.

Cover with lid, bring it to a boil and reduce heat to low. Simmer for 45 to 60 minutes or until the meat is tender and cooked through. If the sauce is not yet thick, cook further without the lid until the desired consistency is achieved.

Transfer the turkey meat into a serving platter, drizzle over with sauce and serve immediately.

Nutritional information per serving: Kcal: 125, Protein: 13.6g, Carbs: 17.3g, Fats: 8.2g

10. Thai Beef Curry with Lime

Ingredients:

2 lb of beef chuck steak, sliced into thin strips

2 tbsp of olive oil

2 tbsp lime leaves, thinly sliced

1 cup of milk, unsweetened

½ cup beef stock or water (optional)

3 tsp of sugar

1 tsp of salt

1 tsp of black pepper, ground

¼ cup of Panang curry paste

Preparation:

Preheat one tablespoon of olive oil in a stew pot over a medium-high temperature. Breafly add one tablespoon of lime leaves.

Add in the curry paste, reduce tempreature to low and cook for about 3 minutes or until aromatic.

Add the meat and cook for 5 minutes while stirring occasionally.

Stir in the sugar, pour in the stock, and milk. Briefly stir to evenly distribute the ingredients and cover with lid. Bring it to a boil and reduce heat to low. Simmer for 30 to 35 minutes or until the beef is tender and cooked through.

Adjust taste and cook further to adjust the consistency of sauce.

Portion the beef curry into individual serving bowls or transfer into a serving bowl and serve immediately.

Nutritional information per serving: Kcal: 425, Protein: 21.2g, Carbs: 18.9g, Fats: 23.2g

11. Ground Cumin Tuna Steaks

Ingredients:

¼ cup of chopped fresh coriander leaves

2 garlic cloves, minced

2 tbsp of lemon juice

½ cup of olive oil

4 tuna steaks

½ tsp of smoked paprika

½ tsp of cumin, ground

½ tsp of chili powder

¼ cup of fresh mint

Preparation:

Add the coriander, garlic, paprika, cumin, chilli powder and lemon juice in a food processor and pulse to combine. Gradually add in the oil and pulse the ingredients until a smooth mixture is achieved.

Transfer the mixture into a bowl, add the fish and gently toss to coat the fish evenly with sauce. Chill for at least 2 hours to allow the flavors to penetrate into the fish.

Remove the fish from the chiller and preheat the gas/charcoal grill. Lightly brush the grid with oil, place the fish and grill for about 3 to 4 minutes on each side.

Remove the fish from the grill, transfer on a serving plate and serve with fresh mint leaves.

Nutritional information per serving: Kcal: 187, Protein: 29.2g, Carbs: 3.4g, Fats: 4.2g

12. Green Bean Burritos

Ingredients:

1 cup of green beans, pre-cooked

1 lb of lean ground beef

1 cup of cottage cheese, crumbled

½ cup of medium-sized onions, finely chopped

1 tsp of red pepper, ground

1 tsp of chili powder

6 whole grain tortillas

Preparation:

Cook up the meat and rinse it. Chop it into bite size pieces and put it back in the pan. Add ground red pepper, chili powder and onions. Stir well for 15 minutes. Remove from the heat.

Combine cottage cheese with green beans in a blender. Mix well for 30 seconds. Add the cheese mixture to the meat. Divide this mixture into 6 equal pieces and spread over tortillas. Wrap and serve.

Nutritional information per serving: Kcal: 248, Protein: 2.4g, Carbs: 7.4g, Fats: 2.1g

13. Egg and Avocado Puree

Ingredients:

4 free-range eggs

1 cup of skim milk

½ avocado, peeled, pit removed, chopped

1 tsp of salt

Preparation:

Gently place two eggs in a pot of boiling water. Cook for 10 minutes. Rinse and drain. Cool for a while and peel. You can add one teaspoon of baking soda in a boiling water. This will make the peeling process much easier. Cut the eggs into bite-sized pieces and refrigerate for about 30 minutes.

Place avocado chops and eggs into the blender. Season with salt to taste. Add milk and blend for 30 seconds or until smooth. This puree should be eaten right away.

Nutritional information per serving: Kcal: 221, Protein: 9.8g, Carbs: 9.5g, Fats: 18.2g

14. Creamy Strawberry Salad

Ingredients:

½ cup of walnuts, ground

2 cups of fresh strawberries, chopped

1 tbsp of strawberry syrup

2 tbsp of whipping cream

1 tbsp of brown sugar

Preparation:

Wash and cut the strawberries into small pieces. Mix with ground walnuts in a bowl. In a separate bowl, combine strawberry syrup, non fat cream and brown sugar. Beat well with a fork and use to top the salad.

Nutritional information per serving: Kcal: 223, Protein: 12.3g, Carbs: 10.2g, Fats: 4.8g

15. Ginger Eggs

Ingredients:

3 free-range eggs

2 tbsp of olive oil

1 tsp of fresh ginger, grated

¼ tsp of black pepper, ground

¼ tsp of sea salt

Preparation:

Beat the eggs with a fork. Add ginger and pepper. Mix well and fry in olive oil for few minutes. Serve warm. Season with sea salt.

Nutritional information per serving: Kcal: 102, Protein: 13.7g, Carbs: 9.5g, Fats: 5.6g

16. Buckwheat Chia Bread

Ingredients:

3 cups of buckwheat flour

3 egg whites

1 cup of chia seeds, minced

1 tsp of salt

½ pack of dry yeast

Warm water

Preparation:

Mix flour, eggs and chia seeds with salt and yeast. Add warm water and stir until smooth dough. Let it stand in a warm place for about 30-40 minutes.

Spread some flour on a working surface. This will prevent the dough from sticking. Now shape the bread using your hands. I always like to shape round breads, but this is not necessary.

Sprinkle with cold water and bake in preheated oven, at 350 degrees for about 40 minutes.

Nutritional information per serving: Kcal: 131, Protein: 6.8g, Carbs: 16.3g, Fats: 4.2g

17. Warm Bean Salad

Ingredients:

14oz of beans, pre-cooked

7oz sweet corn

1 tsp of chili powder

1 tbsp of chopped parsley

3 tbsp of oil

1 medium-sized onion, peeled and chopped

Preparation:

Heat up the oil over a medium temperature. Stir-fry the onion for a couple of minutes. Add chili pepper and about two tablespoons of water and continue to cook for ten more minutes.

Now add the beans, corn, and about ¼ cup of water. Bring it to a boil and cook for another ten minutes. Remove from the heat and transfer to a bowl.

Add chopped parsley and toss to combine. Serve.

Nutrition information per serving: Kcal: 121 Protein: 36g, Carbs: 30.8g, Fats: 14g

18. Cottage Cheese Chia Patee

Ingredients:

½ cup of chia seeds powder

¼ cup of chia seeds

½ cup of cottage cheese, crumbled

¼ cup of parsley, finely chopped

¼ cup of skim milk

1 tbsp of mustard

¼ tsp of salt

Preparation:

Combine parsley and mustard in a mixing bowl and set aside.

Meanwhile, combine cottage cheese with milk, salt, chia seeds powder and chia seeds. Mix well, add parsley and mustard mixture. Allow it to stand in the refrigerator for about an hour before serving

Nutritional information per serving: Kcal: 131, Protein: 14.8g, Carbs: 10.3g, Fats: 7.4g

19. Sunflower Chicken Salad

Ingredients:

3 chicken breast, skinless and boneless, halved

1 cup of Iceberg lettuce, torn

5 cherry tomatoes, halved

2 tbsp of sour cream

1 tbsp of olive oil

1 tsp of fresh parsley, chopped

1 tbsp of sunflower oil

1 tsp of chili pepper, ground

1 tbsp of lemon juice

1 tsp of salt

Preparation:

Cut the chicken breast halves into bite-sized pieces. Mix the sunflower oil, chopped parsley, minced chili pepper, and lemon juice to make a marinade. Put the chicken cubes on a baking sheet, sprinkle with chili marinade and bake at 350 degrees for about 30 minutes. Remove from the oven.

Meanwhile, mix cherry tomatoes with chopped lettuce and low fat cream. Add chicken cubes and season with salt and olive oil.

Toss to combine and serve.

Nutritional informations per serving: Kcal: 282, Protein: 29.4g, Carbs: 9.8g, Fats: 12.3g

20. Creamy Green Beans

Ingredients:

1 cup of green beans, pre-cooked

1 medium-sized tomato, chopped

1 ½ cup of cottage cheese

1 tsp of garlic sauce

1 tbsp of flaxseed oil

1 tsp ofsalt

1 tsp of black pepper, ground

Preparation:

You should buy pre-cooked beans for this one as it will save you some time. If, however, you choose to cook beans yourself, soak them overnight, rinse, and drain before cooking. Place in a deep pot and add enough water to cover.

Cook for 35-40 minutes over medium-high heat. Drain and chill for a while.

Meanwhile, finely chop tomato and palce in a bowl. Add other ingredients and toss well to combine. Season with salt and pepper. Serve cold.

Nutritional informations per serving: Kcal: 192, Protein: 11.3g, Carbs: 20.5g, Fats: 8.7g

21. Baby Spinach and Egg Salad

Ingredients:

4 large eggs, boiled

1 medium-sized carrot, grated

1 cup of baby spinach, chopped

1 tbsp of fresh ginger, grated

1 tbsp of lemon juice

1 tbsp of olive oil

1 tsp of turmeric, grated

1 tsp of salt

Preparation:

Boil the eggs for about 10-12 minutes, remove from heath, peel and cut into small cubes. Place in a large bowl and combine with spinach, grated carrot, and ginger.

Sprinkle with lemon juice, and season with olive oil, turmeric, and salt. Serve cold.

Nutritional informations per serving: Kcal: 97, Protein: 13.3g, Carbs: 4.5g, Fats: 3.5g

22. Red Cabbage with Feta

Ingredients:

1 cup of red cabbage, grated

½ cup of carrots, grated

½ cup of beetroot, grated

1 cup of feta cheese

3 tbsp of almonds, minced

1 tbsp of almond extract

1 tbsp of vegetable oil

1 tsp of salt

Preparation:

Mix the vegetables in a large bowl. Add feta cheese, minced almonds and almond extract. Season with almond oil and salt.

You can add some lemon juice or vinegar, but that is optional.

Nutritional informations per serving: Kcal: 98, Protein: 5.8g, Carbs: 7.2g, Fats: 8.5g

23. Mediterranean Fish Balls

Ingredients:

1½ lbs white fish, boneless

1 tsp of black pepper, freshly ground

½ lb of shrimps

½ lemon juice

1½ cup of almond flour

2 tbsp of tartar sauce

½ cup water

3 tbsp of fresh parsley, finely chopped

3 large eggs

1 tsp of salt

Cooking spray

Preparation:

Use a food processor to make a paste combining 2 eggs, ½ cup almond flour, shrimps, white fish, parsley, and lemon juice, blending till the paste is smooth. Take a bowl, pour some water and break an egg into it. Whisk the two and create a mixture. In a separate bowl, put the remaining almond flour and add salt and pepper to it.

Take a larger bowl and mix the contents of all three bowls. Then, make small balls out of the batter you have created. Put the balls in the skillet and fry for about 15 minutes. Enjoy with tartar sauce.

Nutritional information per serving: Kcal: 54, Protein: 5.2g, Carbs: 4.7g, Fats: 2.5g

24. Butter Shrimps

Ingredients:

2 lbs of large shrimps, peeled and deveined

2 tbsp lemon juice

1 tsp Cayenne pepper, ground

½ tsp of black pepper, ground

1 tsp of sea salt

4 garlic cloves, minced

3 tbsp of butter

2 tbsp of fresh parsley, chopped

2 tbsp of cooking fat

Preparation:

Preheat a large skillet over a medium-high temperature. Add some butter, and cook until melts.

Now, add in the shrimps. Fry the shrimps till almost opaque in appearance.

Add the rest of the ingredients to the skillet. Reduce the heat to low and cook for 30 minutes more.

Nutritional informations per serving: Kcal: 104, Protein: 19.6g, Carbs: 4.8g, Fats: 11.7g

25. Parsley with Nuts & Dates Salad

Ingredients:

2 cups of Italian parsley, roughly chopped

¼ cup of almonds, halved

½ cup of dates, pit removed and halved

2 tbsp of balsamic vinegar

2 tbsp of olive oil

½ tsp of salt

½ tsp of black pepper, ground

Preparation:

Combine the oil, vinegar, salt, and pepper in a small mixing bowl. Whisk well and set aside.

In large salad bowl, combine parsley, almonds, and dates. Toss well and drizzle with dressing.

Refrigerate for 30 minutes before serving.

Nutritional information per serving: Kcal: 58, Protein: 5.2g, Carbs: 10.6g, Fats: 8.7g

26. Soft Cumin Pork Chops

Ingredients:

4 lbs of loin pork chops, trimmed

1 tbsp of brown sugar

1 tsp of salt

1 tsp of chili pepper, ground

For dressing:

1 tsp of cumin, ground

1 tsp of Dijon mustard

½ tsp of smoked paprika, ground

½ tsp of black pepper, ground

1 tbsp of olive oil

Preparation:

Preheat the oil in a large frying skillet over a medium-high temperature.

Meanwhile, combine dressing ingredients in a mixing bowl and set aside.

Place the pork chops into the pan and cook for about 10 minutes from both sides, or until doneness. Reduce the heat to low and cook for 5 minutes more. Remove from the heat and transfer the meat to the serving plate.

Top the meat with dressing.

Serve with some fresh sliced tomatoes. This is, however, optional.

Nutritional information per serving: Kcal: 165, Protein: 24.6g, Carbs: 3.5g, Fats: 12.4g

27. No Bake Coconut Cookies

Ingredients:

2 tbsp of walnuts, roughly chopped

½ small coconut, grated

1 tbsp of Goji berries

1 cup of coconut milk

1tsp of lemon zest

½ tsp of vanilla extract

½ tsp of sugar

1 tsp of cocoa, raw

½ tsp of chili, ground

Preparation:

Combine chili, lemon zest, vanilla extract and coconut milk in a medium deep pot. Cook for about 10 to 15 minutes on a low temperature. Leave it to cool for a while.

Meanwhile, combine walnuts, coconut chops, berries and half cup of water in a food processor. Blend until smooth and transfer to the pot. Give it a final stir to combine.

Use muffin molds to shape cookies. Top with cocoa or grated chocolate and regfigerate for 3 hours before serving.

Nutritional information per serving: Kcal: 135, Protein: 3.2g, Carbs: 10.2g, Fats: 9.4g

28. Parsley Toast

Ingredients:

4 slices of grain bread, whole

½ cup of Mozzarela cheese, crumbled

½ cup of parlsey, finely chopped

2 tbsp of extra virgin olive oil

1 tsp of black pepper, ground

1 tsp of basil, ground

Preparation:

Combine cheese, parsley, and pepper in mixing bowl. Beat well with a fork and set aside.

Spread the olive oil onto bread slices usinga kitchen brush. Place the bread slices in the toaster and set for 2 minutes, or medium toasted.

Spread mixture over the bread slices. Sprinkle with extra teaspoon of ground basil. Eat immediately while warm and crunchy.

You can add a few tomato slices, but this is optional.

Enjoy!

Nutritional information per serving: Kcal: 145, Protein: 8.8g, Carbs: 15.7g, Fats: 5.5g

29. Overnight Pomegranate Oatmeal

Ingredients:

1 cup of oatmeal

½ cup of dried plums, chopped

1 cup of skim milk

1 tbsp of flaxseed

1 tbsp of honey

1 tbsp of pomegranate seeds

1 tbsp of chia seeds

1 tsp of vanilla extract

¼ cup of pomegranate juice

Preparation:

First, combine oatmeal, plums, flaxseed, and vanilla extract in a large mixing bowl. Add milk, honey, pomegranate juice, and stir all well to combine. Top with chia seeds and refrigerate overnight.

Enjoy!

Nutritional information per serving: Kcal: 310, Protein: 12.4g, Carbs: 41.2g, Fats: 9.3g

30. Shrimp Stew with Fire Roasted Tomatoes

Ingredients:

1 cup of fire roasted tomatoes

1 cup of frozen shrimp mix

1 tbsp of dry basil

4 cups fish stock

3 tbsp of tomato paste

3 pieces celery stalks, chopped

3 medium-sized carrots, chopped

2 tbsp of olive oil

1 medium-sized onion, finely chopped

4 garlic cloves, crushed

½ cup of button mushrooms

Preparation:

Heat up the olive oil in a frying pan, over a medium temperature. Add chopped celery, onions, and carrots. Stir well and fry for about 10 minutes.

Remove from the heat and transfer to a deep pot. Add the remaining ingredients and cook for about an hour over a medium temperature. "

Nutritional information per serving: Kcal: 303, Protein: 34.8g, Carbs: 7.4g, Fats: 15.3g

31. Avocado Pancakes

Ingredients:

1 cup of skim milk

1 free-range egg

1 cup of all-purpose flour

½ tsp of salt

1 medium-sized avocado, peeled and pit removed, chopped

½ tbsp of brown sugar

2 tbsp of oil for frying

1 tsp of sugar powder

1 tsp of baking powder

Preparation:

Preheat the oil in a frying skillet over a medium-high temperature.

Meanwhile, combine flour, baking powder, and salt in large mixing bowl. Stir well and add milk and egg.

Stir all well until you get smooth dough mixture. Spoon in mixture into the skillet, and fry until gold brown on both sides. Baked pancakes remove to cool.

Put avocado chops into the food processor. Sprinkle with brown sugar and blend until smooth.

Spread avocado mixture on the pancakes and sprinkle with some sugar powder for decoration.

Serve immediately.

Nutritional information per serving: Kcal: 198, Protein: 7.6g, Carbs: 12.5g, Fats: 12.3g

32. Creamy White Chili

Ingredients:

1 pound of chicken breast, boneless and skinless, cut into ½ inch thick cubes

1 medium-sized onion, peeled and sliced

2 cans of white beans, cooked

1 can of chicken broth

2 cans of green chilies, chopped

3 tbsp of olive oil

Salt and pepper to taste

1 tsp of oregano, dry

1 tsp of cumin, ground

1 cup of sour cream

½ cup of heavy whipping cream

Preparation:

Heat up the olive oil over a medium-high temperature. Add the sliced onions and garlic. Stir-fry for about a minute and add the chicken cubes. Reduce the heat to medium and cook for about 15 minutes.

Add other ingredients, except the sour cream and heavy whipping cream. Mix well and bring it to a boil. Reduce the heat to low, cover and cook for about 30 minutes.

Top with sour cream and heavy whipping cream. Serve warm.

Nutrition information per serving: Kcal: 206 Protein: 45.4g, Carbs: 49g, Fats: 17g

33. Green Tea Smoothie

Ingredients:

3 tbsp of green tea, minced

1 cup of grapes, white

½ cup of kale, finely chopped

1 tbsp of honey

½ tsp of fresh mint, ground

1 cup of water

Preparation:

Combine all ingredients in a blender. Blend until smooth and transfer into the smoothie glasses. Refrigerate 30 minutes before serving.

Serve immediately with some ice cubes.

Nutrition information per serving: Kcal: 301 Protein: 4.8g, Carbs: 55.4g, Fats: 2.1g

34. Thick Chicken Soup

Ingredients:

1 pound of chicken meat, boneless and skinless

1 can of white beans

¼ jalapeno pepper, chopped

1 small onion, peeled and finely chopped

2 garlic cloves, crushed

3 tbsp of vegetable oil

1 tsp of salt

1 tsp of black pepper, ground

2 cups of chicken broth

½ tsp of chili powder

¼ cup of lime juice

½ tsp of cumin, ground

½ tsp of coriander, ground

Preparation:

Rinse and drain the beans. Mash half of the beans with a fork and set aside.

Heat up the oil in a large frying skillet, over a medium temperature. Add garlic, onions and peppers. Stir-fry for several minutes.

Now, add the spices and continue to fry for another minute or two.

Add the beans, chicken meat, chicken broth and lime juice. Bring it to a boil and cook for about 20 minutes.

Add the cliantro and cook for five more minutes. Remove from the heat and let it cool.

Serve!

Nutrition information per serving: Kcal: 118, Protein: 36g, Carbs: 31.8g, Fats: 16g

35. Brussels Sprouts in Tomato Sauce

Ingredients:

3 lbs of oxtail, pre – cooked and boneless

1 ½ lb of brussel sprouts, pre – cooked and drained

1 large red onion

4 garlic cloves

1 tbsp of chili powder

1 large tomato, blended

3 bay leaves

½ cup of fresh parsley, minced

4 cups of water

1 tbsp of olive oil

Preparation:

Pour 6 glasses of water into the pressure pot and add the oxtail. Add 1 tbsp of olive oil and cook for 10 minutes.

Add all vegetables and spices. Water level must cover all ingredients. Add until it is enough. Cook for 45 minutes.

Blend the tomato and transfer mixture into the pressure pot. Cook for more 20 minutes.

Nutritional information per serving: Kcal: 219, Protein: 48.3g, Carbs: 51.4g Fats: 29g

36. Creamy Squid

Ingredients:

1 lb of fresh squid, without the heads

1 cup of cottage cheese

½ cup of Feta cheese

¼ cup of fresh celery,finely chopped"

3 tbsp of olive oil

1 tsp chili pepper, ground

Preparation:

Wash and clean the squid. Pat dry and set aside.

Combine the cottage cheese with Feta cheese, and chopped celery. Mix well and use 1 tbsp of this mixture to fill each squid.

Heat up the olive oil in a large skillet over medium-hight temperature. Fry the squid on each side for several minutes. Remove from the skillet and allow it to cool for about 15 minutes.

Sprinkle with ground chili pepper and serve.

Nutrition information per serving: Kcal: 232, Protein: 24.2g, Carbs: 9.1g, Fats: 10.5g

37. Warm Carrot Soup

Ingredients:

5 large carrots, peeled and sliced

2 tbsp of olive oil

1 cup of cooking cream

2 cups of water

¼ tsp of salt

Preparation:

Heat up the olive oil over a medium temperature. Peel and slice the carrots. Fry for about 15 minutes, stirring constantly.

Reduce the heat, add cooking cream, salt and water. Cook for about 10 minutes.

Nutritional information per serving: Kcal: 115, Protein: 5.8g, Carbs: 16.3g, Fats: 3.4g

38. Warm Vanilla Pudding

Ingredients:

2 cups of milk

½ cup of sugar

2 tbsp of vanilla extract

3 tbsp of cornstarch

1 tbsp of butter

Preparation:

In a medium-sized saucepan, heat the milk until it starts to boil. Meanwhile, combine the sugar with cornstarch and mix well. Pour the mixture into hot milk and mix well. Reduce the heat to minimum and cook until the mixture thickens. Stir in one tablespoon of butter and vanilla extract. Pour into serving glasses and cool well.

Top with chocolate ice cream and some chocolate dessert topping.

Nutritional information per serving: Kcal: 145, Protein: 3.1g, Carbs: 25.2g, Fats: 4.5g

39. Roasted Lamb Chops

Ingredients:

5 lamb loin chops, 1 ½ inch thick sliced

1 cup of vegetable oil

3 garlic cloves, crushed

1 tbsp of fresh thyme leaves, crushed

1 tbsp of fresh rosemary, crushed

1 tbsp of red pepper, ground

1 tsp sea salt

Preparation:

Combine the oil with crushed garlic cloves, fresh thyme leaves, fresh rosemary, red pepper,and salt. Mix well in a large bowl. Add lamb loin chops and turn to coat. Let it stand in the refrigerator for about 2 hours.

Preheat the oven to 350°F.

Place the lamb chops in a large, ovenproof skillet. Add 4 tablespoons of the marinade and reduce the heat to 300°F. Cook for about 15 minutes and remove from the oven.

Now add 4 tablespoons more marinade, turn over the chops, and cook for 15 more minutes.

Remove from the oven and serve with fresh vegetables. Enjoy!

Nutritional information per serving: Kcal: 250, Protein: 26.2g, Carbs: 14.7g, Fats: 5.6g

40. Fresh Lime Salad

Ingredients:

1 cup of lamb's lettuce, chopped

1 large onion, sliced

6-7 medium-sized cherry tomatoes

½ cup of black olives

6-7 medium radishes

½ medium fresh lime, sliced

1 tbsp of fresh lime juice

2 tbsp extra virgin olive oil

½ tsp of salt

Preparation:

Wash and clean the vegetables. Slice the onions and mix with other vegetables in a large

bowl."

Add fresh lime juice, olive oil, and sald. Mix well again. Decorate with lime slices. Enjoy!

Nutritional information per serving: Kcal: 163, Protein: 3.2g, Carbs: 8.7g, Fats: 512.9g

41. Wild Salmon Wraps

Ingredients:

1lb of wild salmon, minced

1 tbsp of mixed vegetable seasoning

1 cup chopped onion

2 tbsp of red pepper, ground

½ cup of tomato puree

8 large Iceberg lettuce leaves

½ cup of shredded cheddar cheese

1 tbsp of vegetable oil

½ cup of chicken stock

Preparation:

Heat up some oil in a non-stick pan over medium-high temperature. Add the salmon meat and cook for 5 minutes, stirring constantly. Stir in the vegetable seasoning, onions, bell pepper and tomato puree and cook it for 5 minutes.

Pour in the water or stock, cover with lid and bring it to a boil. Reduce the heat to low and simmer for about 20 minutes, or until the liquid has reduced in half. Remove the pan from heat and set it aside.

Prepare the lettuce leaves and place them on a work surface. Portion the meat into the 6 to 8 lettuce leaves. Add cheddar cheese and wrap.

Nutritional information per serving: Kcal: 250, Protein: 21.2g, Carbs: 0.5g, Fats: 18.2g

42. Mushrooms with Tomato Sauce

Ingredients:

1 cup of button mushrooms

1 large tomato, peeled and chopped

3 tbsp of olive oil

1 tbsp of parley, finely chopped

1 tsp of salt

½ tsp of black pepper, ground

Preparation:

Preheat the oven to 400°F.

Preheat the oil in a frying skillet over a medium-high temperature. Pour in tomato mixture and add one cup of water. Redice the heat to low and cook for 15 minutes until water evaporates.

Meanwhile, combine tomato, parsley, and salt into blender. Blend until smooth and set aside.

Wash and drain mushrooms and place into the large baking sheet. Spread the sauce over and sprinkle some pepper to taste.

Bake for 10-15 minutes. Remove from the oven and leave it to cool for while.

Serve with sour cream or Greek yogurt. However, this is optional

Enjoy!

Nutritional information per serving: Kcal: 250, Protein: 26.2g, Carbs: 14.7g, Fats: 5.6g

43. Guava Smoothie

Ingredients:

1 cup of guava, seeds removed, chopped

1 cup of baby spinach, finely chopped

1 banana, peeled and sliced

1 tsp of fresh ginger, grated

½ medium-sized mango, peeled and chopped

2 cups of water

Preparation:

Combine all ingredients in a blender. Blend until smooth and transfer to a serving glasses. Refrigerate for 30 minutes before serving.

Enjoy!

Nutritional information per serving: Kcal: 242, Protein: 6.7g, Carbs: 57.4g, Fats: 1.1g

44. Blue Cheese and Bean Dip

Ingredients:

2oz of butter

1 small onion, peeled and chopped

2 garlic cloves, crushed

8.8oz (1 can) of chili beans, pre-cooked

3.5 oz blue cheese, grated

1 tsp of salt

½ cup of water

½ tsp of chili powder

Preparation:

Melt the butter over a medium temperature. Add the onions, crushed garlic, and stir-fry for several minutes, or until nice light brown color.

Add the chili beans and grated cheese. Mix well and cook until the cheese melts. Remove from the heat and chill for a while. Transfer to a blender and mix well for 30 seconds.

Add chili powder and some salt to taste. Mix well and serve.

Nutrition information per serving: Kcal: 71, Protein: 4.3g, Carbs: 17.5g, Fats: 9.1g

45. Turkey and Veal Braid

Ingredients:

2 lbs of turkey breasts,boneless and skinless

1 lb of veal steak, boneless

¼ cup of vegetable oil

1 tsp red pepper, ground

1 tsp of sea salt

Preparation:

Wash and pat dry the meat. Slice the meat into ½ inch thick slices and pound each slice with a mallet. Using a sharp knife, cut the meat slices into 3 equal pieces. Secure the upper part with a toothpick, and braid.

Combine the vegetable oil with red pepper and salt. Spread this mixture over your braids using a kitchen brush. Allow it to stand for about 15 minutes.

Meanwhile, preheat the grill pan over a medium temperature. You can add 1 teaspoon of the marinade in your pan, but that is not necessary.

Fry the braids for about 10 minutes on each side, or until a nice golden color.

Nutritional information per serving: Kcal: 233, Protein: 29.3g, Carbs: 0.2g, Fats: 13.4g

46. Stuffed Bell Pepper Salad

Ingredients:

3 large red bell peppers, whole

1 cup of Feta cheese, crumbled

3 egg whites

3 tbsp sour cream

½ cup of fresh parsley, finely chopped

Preparation:

Wash and clean the bell peppers. Cut off the tops and remove the ribs and seeds. Rinse well. Sprinkle the inside of each bell pepper with some olive oil. Set aside.

Combine the Feta cheese, egg whites, sour cream, and fresh parsley in a bowl. Mix well. Fill the peppers with the Feta mixture.

Serve.

Nutritional information per serving: Kcal: 185, Protein: 11.3g, Carbs: 6.2g, Fats: 13.4g

47. Creamy Mac & Cheese

Ingredients:

1 cup of rice macaroni

½ cup of button mushrooms, sliced

1 small tomato,peeled and chopped

¼ tsp of oregano, ground

½ tsp of brown sugar

2 tbsp Parmesan cheese

2 tbsp of sour cream

2 tbsp of Feta cheese, crumbled

¼ tsp of salt

2 tbsp of olive oil

Preparation:

Boil 3 cups of water in a deep pot. Remove from the heat and place the rice macaroni in it. Let it stand for several minutes. Rice macaroni will soften very quickly so be careful with this. Remove from the pot and drain. Set aside.

Preheat the olive oil over a medium temperature. Finely chop the tomato and fry for about 5 minutes stirring constantly. Add sliced mushrooms, oregano, sugar, and about 1/5 cup of water. Cook for about 10 more minutes. Remove from the heat and add macaroni. Mix well.

Melt the Feta cheese over a minimum temperature. Add sour cream and Parmesan cheese.Mix well. You can add some milk if the mixture is too thick (about 1/4 cup will be enough).

Serve macaroni with tomatoes and mushrooms and pour with cheese mixture.

Nutritional information per serving: Kcal: 180, Protein: 6.8g, Carbs: 22.2g, Fats: 7.3g

48. Cherry Tomatoes Rice

Ingredients:

1 cup brown rice

6 large cherry tomatoes

1 cup button mushrooms

1 tsp dried rosemary, finely chopped

1/8 tsp of salt

3 tbsp of olive oil

Preparation:

Use a package instructions to prepare the rice. Set aside.

Heat up the olive oil in a large skillet. Finely chop the tomatoes and fry for about 10 minutes stirring constantly.

Add the mushrooms and fry until all the water evaporates. Now add dry rosemary and salt.

Mix the tomato sauce with the rice and serve.

Nutritional information per serving: Kcal: 255, Protein: 6.1g, Carbs: 48.4g, Fats: 4.3g

49. Warm Dip Tortillas

Ingredients:

8 tortillas

11oz of grated Gouda cheese

4 spring onions, finely chopped

5.6oz can corn

2 tbsp of oil

For chili dip:

3 large ripe tomatoes

1 tbsp of butter (can be replaced with olive oil)

1 tbsp of ground chili

2 chili peppers, finely chopped

2 garlic cloves, crushed

½ tsp of dry oregano

¼ tsp of salt

1 tsp of sugar

¼ cup of white wine

Preparation:

Heat up a grill pan over a medium-high temperature. Heat each tortilla for about one minute in a microwave. This will make a wrapping process much easier. Spread the gouda over each tortilla and add spring onions, corn and some salt. Wrap and grill each tortilla for about 1-2 minutes on each side, or until the cheese melts. Transfer to a serving platter.

Dip:

Peel and roughly chop the tomatoes. Make sure you keep all the liquid.

Melt the butter over a medium temperature. Add the garlic and stir-fry for several minutes. Now add tomatoes, oregano, salt, sugar, ground chili and finely chopped chili peppers. Reduce the heat to low and cook until the tomatoes have softened. Add wine and cook for 10 more minutes stirring constantly. Serve with tortillas.

Nutrition information per serving: Kcal: 86 Protein: 4.4g, Carbs: 11.5g, Fats: 6.7g

50. Creamy Pide

Ingredients:

½ cup of grated gouda

½ cup of shredded mozzarella

¼ cup of parmesan cheese

½ cup of tomato pizza sauce

1 tsp of dry oregano

1 tbsp of extra virgin olive oil

1 pide bread

Preparation:

Preheat the oven to 350 degrees.

Spread the cheese over pide bread and sprinkle with some dry oregano and olive oil. Bake for 10 minutes, or until the cheese melts. Serve warm!

Nutrition information per serving: Kcal: 369, Protein: 30.2g, Carbs: 58.4g, Fats: 24.2g

ADDITIONAL TITLES FROM THIS AUTHOR

70 Effective Meal Recipes to Prevent and Solve Being Overweight: Burn Fat Fast by Using Proper Dieting and Smart Nutrition

By

Joe Correa CSN

48 Acne Solving Meal Recipes: The Fast and Natural Path to Fixing Your Acne Problems in Less Than 10 Days!

By

Joe Correa CSN

41 Alzheimer's Preventing Meal Recipes: Reduce or Eliminate Your Alzheimer's Condition in 30 Days or Less!

By

Joe Correa CSN

70 Effective Breast Cancer Meal Recipes: Prevent and Fight Breast Cancer with Smart Nutrition and Powerful Foods

By

Joe Correa CSN

www.ingramcontent.com/pod-product-compliance
Lightning Source LLC
Chambersburg PA
CBHW062147020426
42334CB00020B/2544